Diana Isabella Dmytrow

Study: Frequency of simultaneous application of CYP3A inhibitors

Diana Isabella Dmytrow

Study: Frequency of simultaneous application of CYP3A inhibitors

ScienciaScripts

Imprint

Cover image: www.ingimage.com

This book is a translation from the original published under ISBN 978-3-639-63086-2.

Publisher:
Sciencia Scripts
is a trademark of
Dodo Books Indian Ocean Ltd. and OmniScriptum S.R.L publishing group

120 High Road, East Finchley, London, N2 9ED, United Kingdom
Str. Armeneasca 28/1, office 1, Chisinau MD-2012, Republic of Moldova, Europe
Managing Directors: Ieva Konstantinova, Victoria Ursu
info@omniscriptum.com

Printed at: see last page
ISBN: 978-620-8-56496-4

Table of contents

1. Introduction

1.1 Problem definition

Since hospitalized patients usually have comorbidities that require treatment, they receive several medications (AM) at the same time. An AM is released, absorbed, distributed, metabolized and eliminated in the body through the pharmacokinetic LADME process. The application of several AMs can lead to interactions, as the AMs can compete with each other. The focus of this study is the metabolization of AM. AMs can interact in the liver if they are applied simultaneously, as the metabolization process can be inhibited or induced. This happens because only one AM at a time is metabolized by the enzyme in the liver. The other AM, which is applied simultaneously, cannot be metabolized because the enzyme is busy metabolizing the first AM. As a result, the active substance or its metabolite from the second AM circulates in the bloodstream over an unplanned, longer period of time and can therefore cause toxic conditions in patients due to the AM inhibitors. In contrast, the effect of the AM is attenuated with simultaneous application of AM inducers, as the active substance is metabolized faster than intended. This in a loss of efficacy of the AM, as the therapeutic range of the plasma concentration is not reached. In principle, AM interactions are often given little attention due to the lack of time in routine clinical practice, resulting in potential drug-induced toxicity or risks for the patient. As a result, patients may suffer one or more predictable harms that have been avoided. The focus of this study is on cytochrome P-3A (CYP3A) inhibitors because this subgroup represents the largest proportion of the cytochrome P-450 (CYP-450) enzyme family and thus metabolizes most AM.

1.2 Scientific questions

What is the absolute and relative frequency of simultaneously applied CYP3A inhibitors in the clinical routine of inpatients in a hematology and oncology department of a hospital in Germany? What is the relative proportion of patients who are exposed to CYP3A inhibitor interactions?

1.3 Aim of the study

The aim of this study is to empirically investigate the relative frequency of simultaneously applied CYP3A inhibitors in clinical routine, using the example of a Frankfurt hospital, in order to determine the need for intervention in this regard. If the result is significant that CYP3A inhibitors are frequently applied simultaneously, it would make sense to use interaction warning systems from AM. The establishment of a digital interaction warning in an electronic patient record could prevent the simultaneous application of CYP3A inhibitors and protect patients from avoidable, undesirable AM interactions.

2. State of the art

In routine clinical practice, many AMs are administered simultaneously, as inpatients are usually multimorbid. In contrast, AM interactions in therapy combinations have a desirable effect if the AM are coordinated with each other (Hafner et al. 2010). These therapy combinations are frequently used in cytostatic therapy for hematologic and oncologic patients. However, the undesirable AM interactions should be avoided in routine clinical practice, as drug effects can be weakened or intensified and a drug-induced loss of efficacy or drug-induced toxicity can occur (Hafner et al. 2010). 20% of drug effects are adverse drug reactions, which are potentially dangerous and can lead to death (Mutschler 2012, p. 95). A risk assessment is therefore essential. A drug interaction implies an undesirable interaction in which the probability of occurrence increases exponentially with the number of AMs (Mutschler 2012, p. 95). Studies show that patients take at least 3-9 different AMs per day, which entails a high risk of AM interactions (Mutschler 2012, p. 95). This refers to the high number of AMs that patients take or are administered daily. Whether an AM interaction occurs depends on the simultaneously administered AMs. AM incompatibilities often occur excorporeally and can be induced physically, chemically and physico-chemically (Mutschler 2012, p. 95). The biochemical degradation of an active substance is related to the concentration of the AM in the blood and thus in the tissues that metabolize the AM (Lüllmann et al. 2010, p. 56). The enzyme CYP-450 is found in organs such as the lungs, liver, intestine and nose (Horton 2008, p. 214). The mixed-function CYP-450 enzyme degrades a large number of AMs and forms the top group of specific enzymes that metabolize AMs (Lüllmann et al. 2010, p. 56). As many AMs are metabolized by the CYP 450 enzyme, simultaneous application of these AMs leads to known undesirable interactions, as the AMs are metabolized by the same CYP 450 enzyme (Horton 2008, p. 214). This means that the CYP-450 enzyme can only metabolize a single AM at a time. The CYP3A enzyme is a specific subgroup of the CYP-450 enzyme. The metabolization of CYP3A-AM place preferably in the isoenzyme CYP3A of the intestine, the liver, or in the intestine and the liver simultaneously (Wynn et al. 2008, p. 106). When a CYP3A inhibitor AM is applied, the CYP3A enzyme is occupied with its metabolization and cannot metabolize any other AM of the CYP3A class. This results in an increase in the dose in the blood of the other administered AM (Wynn et al. 2008, p. 106). The other simultaneously administered AM, which must also be metabolized via the same isoenzyme, increases the plasma concentration in the bloodstream due to the occupation of the first AM and can thus reach toxic states in the organism with AM inhibitors, as it slows down or blocks the enzyme activity (Mutschler 2012, p. 98). The normal function of the isoenzyme restored when the inhibitor is discontinued or reduced (Greiner 2009, p. 50-51). From the time of discontinuation, inhibitor interactions occur and the toxic states are eliminated.

In the case of CYP inducers, metabolization, i.e. the metabolism of one of the simultaneously administered AMs, is accelerated in the enzyme, as both inducers require the same isoenzyme in order to be metabolized (Mutschler 2012, p. 99). In this case, the drug effect may fail to materialize, as the "therapeutic range" of the plasma concentration of an administered AM not reached (Mutschler 2012, p. 99). The reason for this is the increased provision of the enzyme, which means that more drugs can be metabolized per unit of time (Greiner 2009). To the

"Therapeutic breadth" is illustrated below.

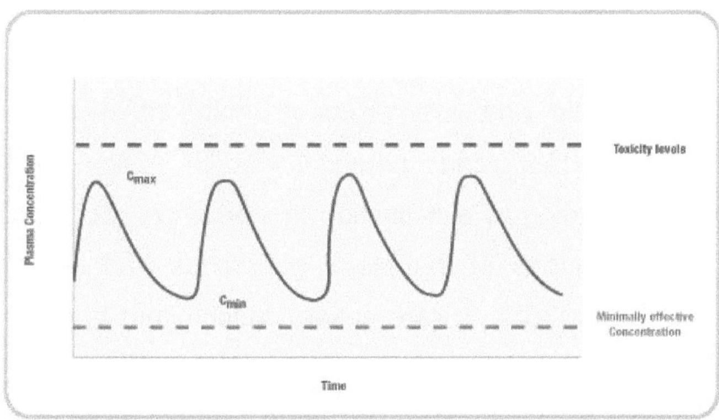

Figure 2.1: Therapeutic range of plasma concentration (Saladax Biomedical Inc. 2014)

The x-axis represents the time, the y-axis the plasma concentration, the C_{max} the maximum plasma concentration and the C_{min} the minimum plasma concentration of an active substance. The therapeutic range begins at the minimum effective concentration and ends directly before the start of the toxic concentration.

Natural substances such as grapefruit can also trigger CYP3A interactions with simultaneous AM application. This is because the grapefruit substance furanocoumarin interacts with many AMs, as it is a CYP3A inhibitor that is metabolized by the intestine and liver (Wynn et al. 2008, p. 113). The use of the grapefruit substance furanocoumarin as a favorable CYP3A inhibitor to achieve dose savings with simultaneous application of other CYP3A inhibitor AMs is dangerous, as only a small time difference means that the therapeutic range of the predicted dose cannot be achieved. The dose of furanocoumarin in grapefruit is subject to natural fluctuations, which is why no exact dose calculations can be made (Wynn et al. 2008, p. 113).

The highly potent CYP3A inhibitors, such as the antifungal AMs ketoconazole and itraconazole and viral protease inhibitors such as ritonavir, may pose important and potential health risks with simultaneous application, leading to a reduction in clearance (CL) and increasing plasma concentrations in the blood (Ioannides and Royal Society of Chemistry 2008, p. 365). In rare cases, concomitant therapy with inhibitory CYP3A-AM such as ketoconazole or erythromycin, which are simultaneously metabolized via CYP3A, has been found to result in a significant concentration of concomitantly administered terfenadine in the bloodstream, which can cause serious and fatal cardiac arrhythmias (Ioannides and Royal Society of Chemistry 2008, p. 365). This interaction can cause serious and fatal cardiac arrhythmias. Simultaneous application of CYP3A inhibitors or other AMs with low therapeutic safety can prolong the QTc interval or cause excessive sedation, rhabdomyolysis or hypotension (calcium channel blockers) (Wynn et al. 2008, p. 111). Despite the predictable adverse interaction effect between CYP3A inhibitors, the drug reaction risk of the patient is not accurately considered in routine clinical practice.

From a scientific and health economic perspective , the CYP3A metabolized AMs represent the most important and most pharmacokinetic AM interactions (Ioannides and Royal Society of Chemistry 2008, p. 365). Furthermore, the CYP3A subfamily is one of the most important of the CYP-450 gene families, as it metabolizes a large number of different AM substance classes via the liver and intestine (Horton 2008, p. 214). As a result, the potency of AM interactions of CYP3A activity, which inhibits or induces the effect, increases (Efferth 2007, p. 24). Pharmacogenetics is presented below, as this represents a further component for influencing metabolization.

2.1. Pharmacogenetics

CYP3A forms a CYP subfamily and has a genetically complex structure, and all humans have significant CYP3A enzyme activity (Wynn et al. 2008, p. 101). There are over 50 different genetic variations that influence the metabolic activity of the CYP3A4 enzyme; two other main enzymes are CYP3A5 and CYP3A7, which are all encoded on chromosome 7 (Wynn et al. 2008, p. 100). Due to the complexity of CYP3A enzymatic activity that the CYP3A subfamily exhibits in genetic variation, it has been clinically determined that CYP3A expression in humans can vary between 10-30-fold (Wynn et al. 2008, p. 101). It has been observed for decades that the metabolization of active substances differs greatly among different ethnicities, as different environmental influences, so-called stressors, influence and change people (Wynn et al. 2008, p. 21). The reason for this is the evolutionary adaptation of metabolization. There are hereditary factors that influence AM metabolism. (Mutschler 2012, p. 106). This variety has a negative on the following ethnicities: Black Africans, Indians and part of the Mediterranean population (Sardinians, Greeks), for example, have a 10% higher probability of suffering hemolytic anemia from the application of metamizole, chloroquine, nitrofurantoin, dapsone and sulfamethoxazole (Mutschler 2012, p. 106). Accordingly, when applying AM, attention must be paid to the ethnicity of the patient in order to avoid this undesirable side effect.

People normally have two copies of a gene, these are called alleles (wild type) (Greiner 2009, p. 51). Genetic polymorphisms occur when variations of this wild type are present; the generic term for this subject area is pharmacogenetics (Greiner 2009, p. 51). Polymorphisms are missing or additional alleles caused by base pair changes, these are called mutations (Greiner 2009, p. 51). There are 3 different metabolization types. The "poor metabolizers" have an allele that is missing or non-functional, so metabolism is greatly reduced in these people. Those affected can only eliminate metabolized substances very slowly (Greiner 2009, p. 51). In contrast, the "ultrarapid (ultraextensive) metabolizers" require more drug than the general population in order to achieve a therapeutic effect (Greiner 2009, p. 51). These people have multiple corresponding wild-type alleles (Greiner 2009, p. 51). general public belongs to the "extensive metabolizers" (Greiner 2009, p. 51).

These metabolize the applied AM in the normal period of time. However, the "extensive metabolizers" can be converted into "poor metabolizers" by AM of the CYP inhibitors, although they are not "poor metabolizers" from a genetic point of view (Greiner 2009, p. 51). The ability to break down xenobiotics, such as AM, decreases considerably with age, which is a further factor in metabolization, as the liver volume and its blood flow through the liver is reduced by up to 30% (Greiner 2009, p. 51). It is therefore essential to reduce the dose of AM in older patients.

2.2. CYP3A inhibitors

In this scientific paper, the focus is on CYP3A inhibitors, as this subgroup has the largest proportion of the CYP 450 enzyme family.

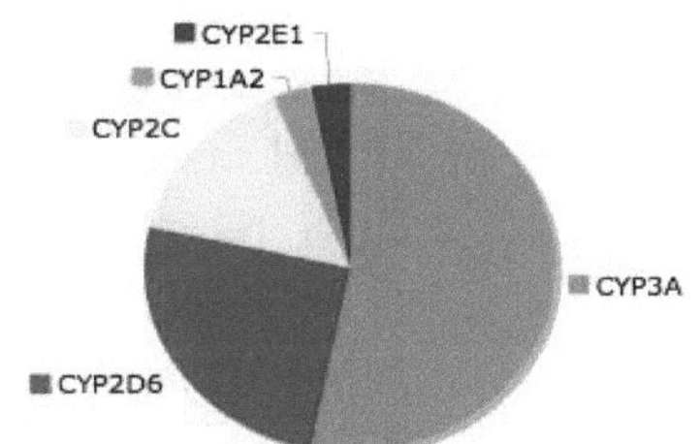

Figure 2.2: Proportion of drug metabolizing CYP-450 enzyme subgroups (Cambridgemedchemconsulting 2012)

The figure the proportions of the CYP-450 subgroups in a pie chart. CYP3A4 the largest proportion, accounting for approx.
takes up >50%. CYP2D6 takes up approx. >25%. CYP2C is approx. >12.5% and the remaining CYP1A2 and CYP2E1 take up the smallest proportions with approx. >4% each.

2.3. CYP3A inhibitor strength

The CYP3A inhibitors are divided into 3 strengths (weak, moderate and strong), which include the following area under the curve (AUC) and CL (U.S. Food and Drug Administration 2011).

Table 2.1: CYP3A inhibitors of strong, moderate and weak strength (U.S. Food and Drug Administration 2011).

Strong inhibitors	**Moderate inhibitors**	**Weak inhibitors**
≥ 5-fold increase in AUC or> 80% decrease in CL	≥ 2 but< 5-fold increase in AUC or 50-80% decrease in CL	≥ 1.25 but< 2-fold increase in AUC or 20-50% decrease in CL

The strengths of the CYP3A inhibitors provide information on the severity of the potential interaction between the AMs. A "strong inhibitor" represents the group of the strongest CYP3A inhibitors and can achieve a ≥5-fold increase in the AM dose in the AUC. The "moderate inhibitors" increase the AUC by≥ 2 to< 5-fold and belong to the group of moderately strong CYP3A inhibitors. An increase in the AUC of ≥ 1.25 to < 2-fold occurs with the "weak inhibitors", which are the weakest CYP3A inhibitors. To illustrate the AUC, an illustration follows:

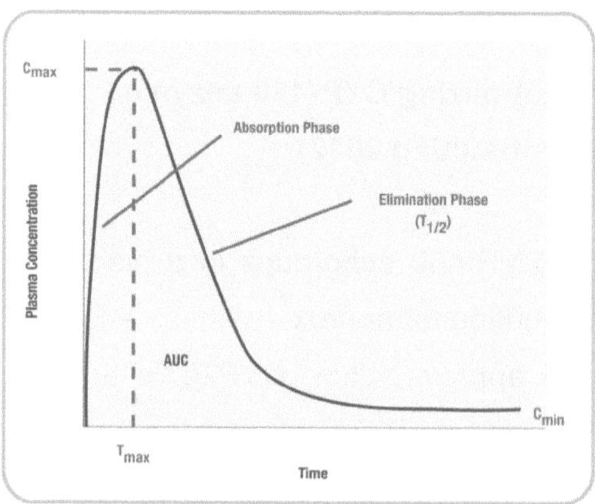

Figure 2.3: AUC in the concentration and time curve (Saladax Biomedical Inc. 2014)

On the Y-axis is the plasma concentration of the applied substance and on the X-axis is the time that has elapsed since the application. C_{max} is the maximum concentration reached and t_{max} is the time in which C_{max} was reached. Two phases are determined on the basis of the curve. The absorption phase begins with uptake and rises to the maximum plasma concentration, the C_{max}. The elimination phase begins after the C_{max} and ends with the lowest plasma concentration, the C_{min}. t½ of the elimination phase is the half-life until 50% of the substance is eliminated from the organism. The total area under the curve is called the AUC. "Area under the Curve" means the area under of the curve (concentration-time curve {amount*time/volume}) of a drug in the bloodstream (Lücker et al. 1982, p. 135). With regard to the table, this means that the plasma concentration is increased more than x-fold by the respective CYP3A inhibitor.

The creatinine CL is used to calculate kidney function, i.e. how well the kidneys can excrete the breakdown products. The "Strong Inhibitor" reduces the CL by at least 80%. This means that the kidney can potentially be damaged by the longer-lasting degradation products of CYP3A inhibitors and therefore the probability of damage must be prevented or taken into account by considering a risk-benefit analysis. The methodology of this study is described below.

3. Methodology

This chapter explains the method to be used in the scientific study "Retrospective empirical study on evaluation of the frequency of simultaneous application of CYP3A inhibitors in clinical routine using the example of a Frankfurt hospital" . Prospective data collection does not represent an advantage over retrospective data collection for this study, because recall and selection bias can also be avoided in retrospective studies. With prospective and pseudonymized data collection, data protection declarations must be obtained from patients, which in turn represents a selection of the sample. There is also no intervention within this study, so prospective data analysis is not advantageous. An empirical, retrospective and anonymized data collection was chosen, which uses inductive and descriptive statistics to evaluate and analyze the data of inpatient records from a Frankfurt hospital. The period evaluation of the patients is carried out retrospectively from the date of approval of the disposition of this scientific work, so that distortions such as recall bias are excluded. Likewise, from the beginning of the evaluation, all patients without exception are considered continuously and the documentation of the patients takes place over the entire inpatient stay, so that no selection bias of the individual days can occur. In terms of content, each AM applied is documented from the patient file with the date of application and the patient's diagnosis. The diagnoses are recorded in this scientific study so that potential correlations with AMs such as CYP3A inhibitors and their interactions can be analyzed. Furthermore, the variety of diagnoses collected in the sample is relevant, as there could be anomalies. These anomalies may be due to chance and therefore not representative, or they may be statistically significant. This needs to be investigated in more detail using statistical tests.

The patient data in the Case Report Form (CRF) is anonymized in accordance with the German Data Protection Act and marked with a consecutive number as an ID. The CRF created in Microsoft Excel by documenting the data from the patient file. The FDA published a list of CYP3A inhibitors with the generic names on its website (U.S. Food and Drug Administration 2011). For this scientific paper, a transcription of the FDA list of CYP3A inhibitors was created for the German trade names, as the documentation of the AM from the patient file is usually done with trade names and thus an optimal comparison can take place (see appendix). The applied AMs are then categorized into the known CYP3A inhibitors and their degree of effectiveness (strong, moderate, weak). The relative frequency of the simultaneously applied CYP3A inhibitors, i.e. the exposed group, is shown below and compared with the non-exposed group. The unexposed group is the group that did not receive any CYP3A inhibitors simultaneously. The data are also analyzed specifically with regard the relative and absolute frequencies of the CYP3A inhibitors applied in single and multiple doses, with their degree of effectiveness (strong, moderate, weak). The patients' diagnoses are examined for abnormalities with regard to the CYP3A inhibitors applied.

Due to the retrospective analysis and the anonymized patient data, no patient information, declaration of consent or data protection declaration is required. An ethics vote is also not required, as there is no medical intervention by the patients, no doctor is involved in the study and the data is collected retrospectively.

3.1 Sample size

The following is the formula for the minimum sample size for discrete data for statements on the population:

$$n = \lceil \left(\frac{z}{\Delta}\right)^2 * \hat{p} * (1 - \hat{p}) \rceil$$

n: The required minimum sample size z: Quantile of the standard normal distribution.

Assumption: The confidence level should be 95%, which means that z = 1.96 (t-table).

Δ: Half the interval width of the measurement accuracy (granularity).

Assumption: The resolution should be ±5%.

$\hat{p}$: The estimated probability that a patient receives two CYP3A inhibitors simultaneously during one day of hospitalization. High probabilities lead to a conservatively high sample size, which is why a high value of 20% is assumed.

If the assumed values are used in the above formula, a minimum sample size of n = 246 is calculated. Within the study, the sample size was adjusted to 315 in order to minimize the statistical error.

1. type to be minimized. Furthermore, larger samples increase the significance of the result (Bortz and Lienert 2008, p. 51). Accordingly 315 data points were analyzed for simultaneous CYP3A inhibitor application . One data point represents one day of a patient's inpatient stay. From a preliminary analysis of the Frankfurt hospital, a patient in the hematology and oncology department is hospitalized for an arithmetic mean of 7 days (Frankfurt Hospital 2015).

3.2 Hypothesis test

As discrete and nominally scaled data are collected within the sample, Pearson's chi-square (χ^2) is suitable as a hypothesis test to check the significance of a difference between two characteristics. In order to test the stochastic independence of the variables, a χ^2 independence test should be carried out. The requirements for atest are met if the variables are nominally scaled, the sample was randomly selected and the expected frequencies are >5 (Bühl 2008, p. 267). Phi coefficient (ϕ) and Cramer's V index (CI) can also be used to examine the effect size of the variables. The ϕ is used to determine the level contingency between two 2-tiered characteristics and the stochastic independence of both variables is tested by the null hypothesis using the significance test ϕ (Bühl 2008, p. 259). The contingency of two alternative characteristics is determined by the ϕ as a measure of correlation (Bühl 2008, p. 271). The generalization of the ϕ represents the CI (Bühl 2008, p. 271). The hypothesis tests are carried out using the IBM SPSS Statistics software. The following hypotheses must be established for the hypothesis test in order to check whether the data are stochastically independent:

Hypotheses

Null hypothesis (H0): The two characteristics are stochastically independent of each other.

Alternative hypothesis (H1): The two characteristics are stochastically interdependent.

The results of the scientific work are presented in the following chapter.

4. Results

The following results were achieved within the study: Data was collected retrospectively from the time of disposition release, 15/09/15, in order to retrospectively observe a period of time that was as random as possible. A patient list from the hospital information system of a Frankfurt hospital was used to chronologically document the drug data and diagnostic data of all patients in a CRF who were admitted to the hematology and oncology department as inpatients during this period. The total number of cases (n) in the sample was adjusted from 246 to 315 in order to make a more precise statement, which is statistically more significant. Accordingly, all medications given were collected on 315 inpatient days from a total of 48 patients between 12.07.15 and 14.09.15 (period 65 days). The longest length of stay of an inpatient was 32 days, the shortest length of stay was 2 days. The arithmetic mean length of stay of an inpatient was 6.5 days and the median was 5 days. In absolute terms, 2383 AM were applied to 48 patients over 315 days, predominantly in the morning at the same time. This results in an arithmetic mean value of 49.65 AM per patient and 7.57 AM per inpatient day.

4.1 Patient characteristics (diagnoses)

The following diagnoses were identified in the 48 inpatients in the sample:

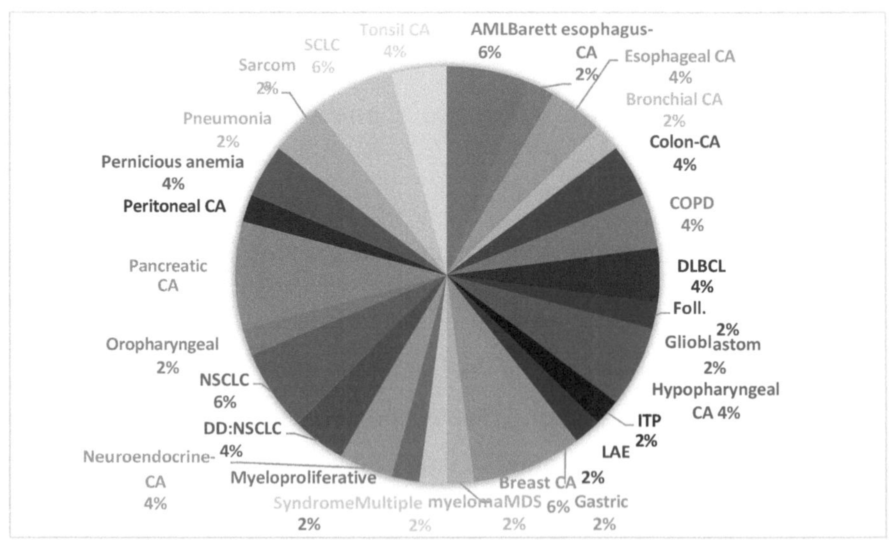

Figure 4.1: Proportion of patients with this diagnosis

The diagnoses of the patients are broadly diversified, with no diagnosis accounting for more than 8% of the sample. Pancreatic carcinoma (CA) patients make up the largest proportion of the sample with 8%, closely followed by acute myeloid leukemia (AML), breast CA, small cell lung cancer (SCLC) and non-small cell lung cancer (NSCLC) with 6% each. The remaining patient diagnoses have smaller proportions. This results in the following proportion of inpatient days for each diagnosis.

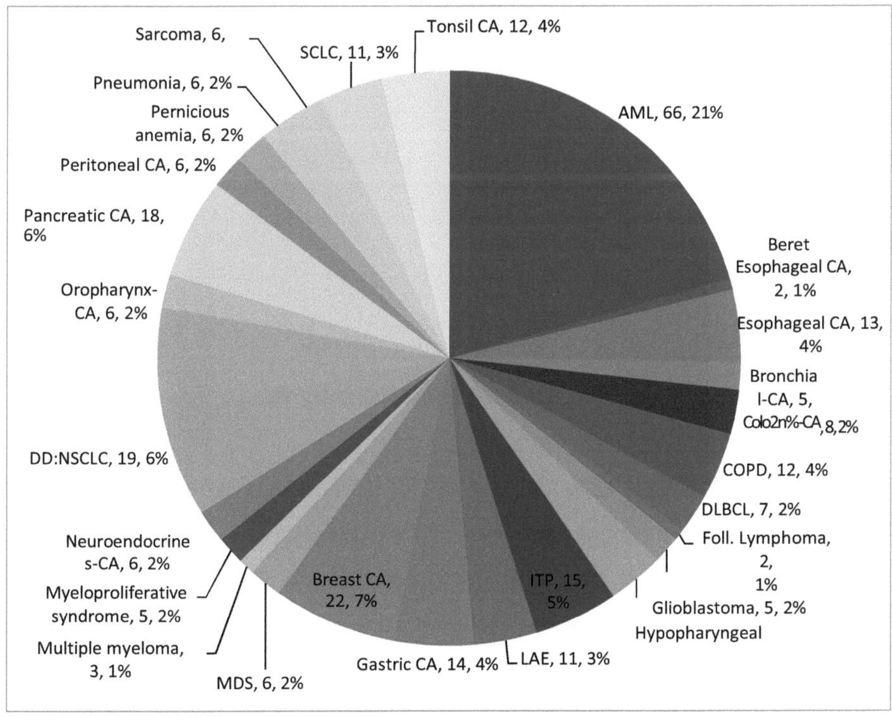

Figure 4.2: Proportion of inpatient days broken down by diagnosis

The diagnoses of all patients were shown in relation to the number of inpatient days. The relative proportion and the absolute frequency of the diagnoses are shown in the pie chart. It can be seen that AML, at 21% (66 of 315 inpatient days), reflects the largest proportion of inpatient stays in this sample. In second place is breast CA with 7% (22/315). NSCLC (19/315), differential diagnostic NSCLC (19/315) and pancreatic CA (18/315) share third place with 6% each.

The following pie chart shows the proportion of diagnoses at for which CYP3A inhibitors were applied simultaneously (on the same day):

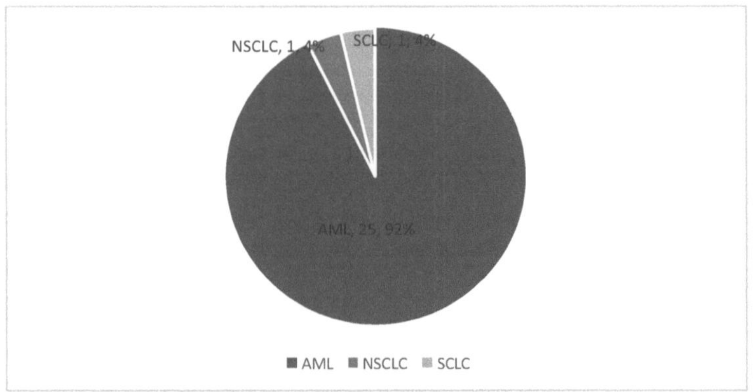

Figure 4.3: Proportion of simultaneously applied CYP3A inhibitors by diagnosis

In the case of AML, 92% (25 out of 27 inpatient days) were diagnosed with simultaneous application of CYP3A inhibitors. NSCLC and SCLC are each at 4% (1 of 27 days). In the remaining 25 of 28 diagnoses in this sample, no CYP3A inhibitors were applied simultaneously.

4.2 Applied medicines

A total of 2383 AMs were applied in this study. The following table the 168 different AMs in alphabetical order. The AM written in red are the applied CYP3A inhibitors, the AM written in black are no CYP3A inhibitors.

Table 4.1: List of drugs applied

5-Fluorouracil	Cernevite	Fortecortin
A&S Inhalation	Cinnarizine, dimenhydrinate	Gemcitabine
Acetylcysteine	Ciprofloxacin	Glycerol trinitrate
Acetylsalicylic acid	Cisplatin	Indacaterol maleate
Adrenaline inhalation	Citalopram	Granisetron
Agomelatine	Clarithromycin	Haloperidol
LFS	Clemastine	Heparin
Algeldrat, magnesium hydroxite	Clopidogrel	Hydrochlorothiazide
Alizapride hydrochloride	Clotrimazole	Hydroxycarbamide
Allopurinol	Codeine	Ibuprofen
Aluminum/magnesium hydroxide, oxetacaine	Colecalciferol	Idarubicin
Amiodarone	Cotrimoxazole	Imepenem
Amlodipine	Cyclophosphamide	Imipenem Carbapeneme
Amphotericin B	Cytarabine	Insulin
Ampicillin	Dabigatran etexilate mesilate	Insulin aspart
Ampicillin Sulbactam	Dexamethasone	Insulin isophane (human)
Aprepitant	Digitalis glycosides	Irinotecan
Atropine	Dimenhydrinate	Isosorbide dinitrate ret
Benperidol	Dimetindene	Potassium
Bisacodyl	Docetaxel	Potassium effervescent
Bisoprolol	Doxepin	hydrogen carbonate,
Budesonide, formoterol	Doxorubicin	Potassium chloride
Butylscopolamine	Dulcolax	Klysma
Calcium folinate	Iron glycine sulfate complex	Lactobacillus ferment
Calcium chloride	Emser salt inhalation	Lactulose
Candecor 32/25	Enoxaparin, sodium salt	Laetrase
Capecitabine	Erlotinib	Laxas
Caphosol mouthwash	Etoposide	Laxoberal
Carbidopa, levodopa 100/25	Etoricoxib	Levetiracetam
Carboplatin	Exemestane	hydrochloride
Carvedilol	Ezetimibe, Simvastatin	Levothyroxine
Cefpodoxime	Fentanyl	Loidocaine
Ceftazidime	Filgrastim	Loperamide
Ceftriaxone	Fondaparinux	Lorazepam
Maaloxan	Pantoprazole	Smofkabives
Macrogol	Paracetamol	Spironolactone
Magnesium Verla	Paracodin	Tamsulosin
Mannitol	Phytomenadione	Tavegil
Marcumar	Piperacillin	Tazobactam, Piperacillin
Mesna	Piracetam	Teicoplanin

Metamizole	polystyrene-co-divinylbenzene)-sulfonic acid, calcium salt	Theophylline
Metformin	Posaconazole	Thiamazole
Metoclopramide	Prednisolone	Platelet concentrate
Metoprolol	Prednisone	Tiotropium bromide
Metronidazole	Pregabalin	Torasemide
Mirtazapine	Pyridoxine h., thiamine nitrate	Tramadol
Morphine	Pyridoxine h., thiamine nitrate S	Tretinoin
Moxofloxacin	Quetiapine hemifumarate	Triazolam
Moxonidine	Ramipril	Valsartan
Nadroparin	Ranitidine	Vancomycin
Oxycodone hydrochloride	Wrestler	vincristine
Sodium picosulfate	Rituximab	Vitamin B12
Nebivolol	Rivaroxaban	Vitamin D3+ Ca
Nifedipine	S&A Inhalation	Voriconazole
Oxazepam	Simeticone	Zinc
Pancreas powder (pig)	Simvastatin	Zopiclone

7 different CYP3A inhibitors were administered within the study. This represents 4.17% of all AMs administered (7 out of 168 drugs). Among these 7 CYP3A inhibitors, the AMs belong to the following strengths:

Table 4.2: Strengths of the 7 different CYP3A inhibitors

Appearance	Strength CYP3A inhibitor
2	A (weak inhibitor)
2	B (moderate inhibitor)
3	C (strong inhibitor)

3 out of 7 CYP3A inhibitors are assigned to strength C. 2 out of 7 CYP3A inhibitors are assigned to strength A and B respectively. This information refers only to the 7 different CYP3A inhibitors in Table 4.1.

A total of 2383 AMs were administered to 48 patients within 315 days. Of these, 2239 applied AM (93.96%) were not CYP3A inhibitors, 43 (1.8%) were weak CYP3A inhibitors (≥ 1.25 but< 2-fold increase in AUC or 20-

50% decrease in CL), 37 (1.55%) moderate CYP3A inhibitors (≥ 2 but < 5- fold increase in AUC or 50-80% decrease in CL) and 64 (2.69%) strong CYP3A inhibitors (≥ 5-fold increase in AUC or > 80% decrease in CL). No AMs were applied on 9 of 315 days. For a better overview, these three categories were "A" (weak), "B" (moderate) and "C" (strong). AMs without a CYP3A inhibiting effect are assigned to category "Z". The following figure shows an overview of the amount of AM applied by category.

Table 4.3: Number of CYP3A inhibitors (weak, moderate, strong) and their proportion in relation to total medicinal products

Total	Number A (weak CYP3A-inhibitor)	Number B (moderate CYP3A-inhibitor)	number C (strong CYP3A-inhibitor)	Number Z (no CYP3A-inhibitor)
Absolute	43	37	64	2239
Share of total pharmaceuticals (2383)	1,80%	1,55%	2,69%	93,96%

There were 43 (1.80%) "weak inhibitors" and 37 (1.55%) "moderate inhibitors",

64 (2.69%) "strong inhibitors" and 2239 (93.96%) AM, which are not CYP3A inhibitors, were applied within the study. The simultaneously applied CYP3A inhibitors are shown below.

4.3 Simultaneously applied CYP3A inhibitors

The following frequencies and their proportions result from the total of 27 days on which CYP3A inhibitors were applied simultaneously:

Table 4.4: Number and proportions of simultaneously applied CYP3A inhibitors in relation to total drugs and days

Number of days of simultaneously applied CYP3A-Inhibitors (all strengths)	Number of days of simultaneously applied CYP3A-Inhibitors between A and B	Number of days of simultaneously applied CYP3A-Inhibitors between A and C	Number of days of simultaneously applied CYP3A-Inhibitors between B and C	Number of days of simultaneously applied CYP3A-Inhibitors between A and A	Number of days of simultaneously applied CYP3A-Inhibitors between B and B	Number of days of simultaneously applied CYP3A-Inhibitors between C and C	
27	1	12	13	1	0	0	**Absolute**
100,00%	3,70%	44,44%	48,15%	3,70%	0,00%	0,00%	**Share**
1,13%	0,04%	0,50%	0,55%	0,04%	0,00%	0,00%	**Share of total appl. Medicinal products (2383)**
8,57%	0,32%	3,81%	4,13%	0,32%	0,00%	0,00%	**Share of total days (315)**

Pharmaceuticals Total	2383	**Days Total**	315	**Total patients**	48

The most frequently simultaneously applied CYP3A inhibitors are of strength B and C (13/27; 48.15%) and A and C (12/27; 44.44%). CYP3A inhibitors of strength B and B (0/27; 0%) and C and C (0/27; 0%) were not applied simultaneously. Only a small number of CYP3A inhibitors of strengths A and A (1/27; 3.7%) and A and B (1/27; 3.7%) were applied simultaneously. If the proportion of simultaneously applied CYP3A inhibitors of the total applied AM of this sample is added up, this results in a value of 1.13% (27 days with 2 simultaneously applied CYP3A inhibitors each of 2383 drugs). The proportion of days of inpatient stay on which at least two CYP3A inhibitors were applied simultaneously was

8.57% (27 days with simultaneously applied CYP3A inhibitors of 315 inpatient days in total). A maximum of only one simultaneous application of two CYP3A inhibitors per day was recorded. The number of CYP3A inhibitors applied is shown below according to their strength weak/moderate/strong, as well as the number of AMs that are not CYP3A inhibitors, divided total, exposed and unexposed patients. The totals and percentages are then calculated.

4.4 Comparison of patients after application of CYP3A inhibitors (total, exposed and non-exposed patients)

In this chapter, the applied CYP3A inhibitors and their strength are compared with the different groups in order to objectively illustrate the differences.

Table 4.5: Total CYP3A inhibitors administered for exposed and unexposed patients

All patients	**Number A** (weak CYP3A inhibitor)	**Number B** (moderate CYP3A-inhibitor)	**Number C** (strong CYP3A inhibitor)	**Number Z** (no CYP3A inhibitor)	**Total**
Absolute	43	37	64	2239	2383
share to total pharmaceuticals	1,80%	1,55%	2,69%	93,96%	100,00%
Exposed patients	**Number A** (weak CYP3A inhibitor)	**Number B** (moderate CYP3A-inhibitor)	**Number C** (strong CYP3A inhibitor)	**Number Z** (no CYP3A inhibitor)	**Total**
Absolute	19	14	47	454	534
proportion to applied drugs	3,56%	2,62%	8,80%	85,02%	100,00%

Non-exposed patients	Number A (weak CYP3A inhibitor)	Number B (moderate CYP3A-inhibitor)	number	Number	Total
Absolute	24	23	17	1785	1849
proportion to applied drugs	1,30%	1,24%	0,92%	96,54%	100,00%

In all 3 groups, the proportion of administered AMs that are not CYP3A inhibitors predominates. For all patients, the proportion of CYP3A inhibitors of strength C is in second place with 2.69%, strength A in third place with 1.80% and strength B in fourth place with 1.55%. It is striking that the total number of AMs applied to unexposed patients (534) is significantly lower than the total number of AMs applied to unexposed patients (1849), which is due to the larger number of unexposed patients. Nevertheless, more type C inhibitors were administered to exposed patients (47) than to unexposed patients (17). There could be a systematic correlation here, which will be investigated in the further course of the study.

4.5 Patients with simultaneously applied CYP3A inhibitors

A total 4 out of 48 (8.33%) patients received simultaneous application of CYP3A inhibitors. The shortest inpatient stay of a patient who received simultaneous CYP3A inhibitors was 2 days. The longest length of stay was 32 days. The other two patients who received simultaneous CYP3A inhibitors were hospitalized for 25 and 3 days respectively. If the 4 patients who received simultaneous CYP3A inhibitors are differentiated, the following values result :

- NSCLC patient: 2 inpatient days, including 1 day with

simultaneous application of CYP3A inhibitors (1/2 = 50%)

- SCLC patient: 3 inpatient days, including 1 day with simultaneous application of CYP3A inhibitors (1/3 = 33.33%)
- AML patient 1: 25 inpatient days, of which 13 days with simultaneously applied CYP3A inhibitors (13/25 = 52%)
- AML patient 2: 32 inpatient days, of which 12 days with simultaneously applied CYP3A inhibitors (12/32 = 37.5%)

summary, this results in an arithmetic mean of 43.21% and a median of 43.75% of the inpatient days on which simultaneous application of CYP3A inhibitors occurred in the exposed patients. The individual diagnoses of the simultaneously applied CYP3A inhibitor patients and the frequency of simultaneously applied CYP3A inhibitors are shown in tabular form below, with differentiation between weak, moderate and strong.

Table 4.6: Number of days of simultaneously applied CYP3A inhibitors (weak, moderate, strong) divided according to the diagnoses of the exposed patients

Diagnosis	Number of simultaneous CYP3A Inhibitors between A and B	Number of simultaneous CYP3A Inhibitors between A and C	Number of simultaneous CYP3A Inhibitors between B and C	Number of simultaneous CYP3A Inhibitors between A and A	Number of simultaneous CYP3A Inhibitors between B and B	Number of simultaneous CYP3A Inhibitors between C and C
NSCLC	1	0	0	0	0	0
SCLC	0	0	0	1	0	0
AML	0	0	13	0	0	0
AML	0	12	0	0	0	0
Total	**1**	**12**	**13**	**1**	**0**	**0**

The NSCLC patient had CYP3A inhibitors of strength A and B administered simultaneously on one day; the SCLC patient had CYP3A inhibitors of strength A and A administered simultaneously on one day. One of the AML patients had CYP3A inhibitors of strength B and C administered simultaneously on 13 days, the other AML patient had CYP3A inhibitors of strength A and C administered simultaneously on 12 days. There was no change in the combination of CYP3A inhibitors administered within the patients during the entire inpatient period. This means that although the combination of CYP3A inhibitors was paused occasionally on inpatient days, the same combination of CYP3A inhibitors was maintained thereafter. There was therefore no change in the combination of CYP3A inhibitors applied. In the exposed AML patients, a "strong inhibitor" was administered with each simultaneous application of the CYP3A inhibitors (only strengths A and C and B and C of the CYP3A inhibitors). The results of the scientific work presented above are critically discussed below.

5. Discussion

In this chapter, the previously evaluated results from the scientific work summarized, critically discussed and the questions answered. The previous calculation of the number of cases was increased from n=246 to n=315 data points in order reduce the statistical error of the first kind. The data collection period was 65 days, a total of 315 inpatient days were analyzed. The planned start of data collection was adhered to, so recall or selection bias can be ruled out, as the disposition release of this study was freely chosen by the scientific management of the study program. Data was collected from 48 patients who were hospitalized at the clinic for an arithmetic mean of 6.5 days. In the preliminary analysis of the Frankfurt hospital, an arithmetic mean inpatient stay of 7 days was observed. Both values are close together, so can speak of a representative sample with regard to the length of inpatient stay, as this study data the reality of clinical routine. If these values were far apart, a non-representative sample could be present and thus a distorted reality could be depicted. 2383 AM were applied over 315 patient days. This results in an arithmetic mean value of 49.65 AM per patient and 7.57 AM per inpatient day. Mutschler (2012) spoke of 3-9 AM per day, cf. chapter 2. The number of AM from this study is therefore within the tolerance range of the result from the previous literature. This is a further that the sample of this study is representative and therefore reflects reality. The individual diagnoses of the patients are discussed below.

5.1 Patient characteristics (diagnoses)

A total of 28 different diagnoses were identified in the patients. The distribution of diagnoses in relation to the number of patients does not show any major differences. This means that the diagnoses are relatively evenly distributed, as in regular clinical routine, and that no dominant diagnosis prevails in the sample. The 5 most common diagnoses are pancreatic CA, AML, breast CA, SCLC and NSCLC. The remaining hematologic and oncologic diagnoses follow closely behind, see Fig. 4.1.

If the proportion of inpatient days is compared with the diagnoses, AML patients account for the largest proportion within the sample at 21%. Breast CA is at 7% and the remaining diagnoses are <7%. Thus, the arithmetic mean inpatient length of stay of 6.5 days is at least 3 times higher for AML diagnoses and therefore deviates significantly from the average.

The CYP3A inhibitors were applied simultaneously in a total of 3 diagnoses in this sample: NSCLC, SCLC and AML. The remaining diagnoses no simultaneous application of CYP3A inhibitors. At 92% (25 of 27 days), AML is the most common diagnosis in which CYP3A inhibitors were administered simultaneously. The proportion is significantly lower for NSCLC and SCLC at 4% each (1 out of 27 days). Based on the results, it can be assumed that AML patients have a higher probability of receiving simultaneous CYP3A inhibitors. However, it must be ruled out that this result is due to chance. To confirm the statistical significance, a χ^2-test of the diagnoses and their inpatient days must be carried out. AML is compared with all other diagnoses (see Chapter 5.6). This is followed by a discussion of the AM applied in this study.

5.2 Applied medicines

A total of 168 different AMs were applied 2383 times on 315 inpatient days. No AMs were administered on 9 out of 315 days. Among all AMs, 7 different CYP3A inhibitors (4.17%) were administered:

Table 5.1: Applied CYP3A inhibitors

Amlodipine (weak CYP3A inhibitor)
Aprepitant (moderate CYP3A inhibitor)
Ciprofloxacin (moderate CYP3A inhibitor)
Clarithromycin (strong CYP3A inhibitor)
Posaconazole (strong CYP3A inhibitor)
Ranitidine (weak CYP3A inhibitor)
Voriconazole (strong CYP3A inhibitor)

This means that only a small proportion of CYP3A inhibitors are administered to inpatients in routine clinical practice. Most of the AMs administered (93.96%) are not CYP3A inhibitors. 1.8% are weak inhibitors, 1.55% are moderate inhibitors and 2.69% are strong inhibitors. Overall, a small proportion of CYP3A inhibitors were administered. The simultaneously applied CYP3A inhibitors are discussed below.

5.3 Simultaneously applied CYP3A inhibitors

In this sample, CYP3A inhibitors were administered simultaneously on 27 out of 315 inpatient days, making interactions between AM possible. This results in an average probability of 8.57% (27 out of 315 days) per inpatient day that a patient is exposed to a simultaneous application. This result answers the questions of this scientific work, cf. chapter 1.1. In the case number planning, an assumption of 20% was made, cf. chapter 3, that CYP3A inhibitors are applied simultaneously to patients per day. In fact, CYP3A inhibitors were administered simultaneously per day in 8.57% of inpatient stays. This results in a difference of 11.43% and indicates that the original planning of the number of cases was too conservative. No comparable study was conducted at the start of the study, so a theoretical assumption had to be made. As the data points (number of cases) were increased by 28.05% during the data evaluation in order to minimize the statistical error of the first kind, a corrective adjustment is to be expected in this respect.

Most of the simultaneously applied CYP3A inhibitors, calculated over the entire 27 days on which CYP3A inhibitors were applied, took place with CYP3A inhibitors of strength B+C (48.15%) and A+C (44.44%). This means that the AUC of strength B increases by≥ 2 to< 5-fold or the CL is reduced by 50-80%. For C, this would be a ≥ 5-fold increase in AUC or a> 80% reduction in CL. For strengths A+A and A+B, the proportion is 3.7%. This means that with the strength A CYP3A inhibitor there is an AUC increase of ≥ 1.25 to < 2-fold or the CL is reduced by 20-50%. This disproportionate increase in the plasma concentration of the active substance or reduction in the excretion of harmful substances by the kidneys can lead to serious side effects that could have been avoided by AM alternatives, see Chapter 2. In order to determine the AM interaction side effect caused by the simultaneous application of CYP3A inhibitors, a further study must be conducted. Here, the adverse events of the patients must be documented and evaluated, namely whether actual interactions have taken place.

5.4 Comparison of the applied CYP3A inhibitors (total, exposed and unexposed patients)

The results in Table 4.7 show that the AMs of non-CYP3A inhibitors predominate in the total, exposed and non-exposed patients, but that the strong inhibitors were applied second most frequently in the total and exposed patients. In non-exposed patients, the weak inhibitors were the second most frequently applied CYP3A inhibitors. The conclusion from this table is that, in principle, most AMs in this sample are not CYP3A inhibitors and that when CYP3A inhibitors were used, they were mostly of strength C (strong inhibitors). This result also shows that most CYP3A inhibitors were administered to the exposed patients.

5.5 Patients with simultaneously applied CYP3A inhibitors

The proportion of non-CYP3A inhibitor AM was highest in the exposed patients who were simultaneously administered CYP3A inhibitors in the study period, at 85.02%. CYP3A inhibitors of strength C accounted for 8.8% of the AM administered, followed by inhibitors of strength A with 3.56% and finally strength B with 2.62%. This means that CYP3A inhibitors of strength C were administered most frequently, namely by >50% more frequently than the other two strengths. Since strength C is the strong inhibitor and causes a≥ 5-fold increase in AUC or >80% reduction in CL, it is recommended that AM combinations be reconsidered in this respect in order to protect patients toxicity. It is also striking that the combination of CYP3A inhibitors was retained in all cases. Accordingly, there was no change in the combination of CYP3A inhibitors applied. This is probably a systematic administration of specific AMs in combination. If the AMs were better coordinated to avoid interactions, the risk to the patient could be avoided with little effort.

To summarize the results, a small proportion of 8.33% (4 of 48) of patients received simultaneous application of CYP3A inhibitors and thus potentially suffered CYP3A inhibitor interactions. This result also answers the questions relating to the absolute and relative frequency of simultaneous application of CYP3A inhibitors in clinical routine. The data analysis reveals an above-average frequency of simultaneously applied CYP3A inhibitors, particularly in the diagnosis of AML. No such accumulation was found for the other diagnoses. The following figure illustrates this fact:

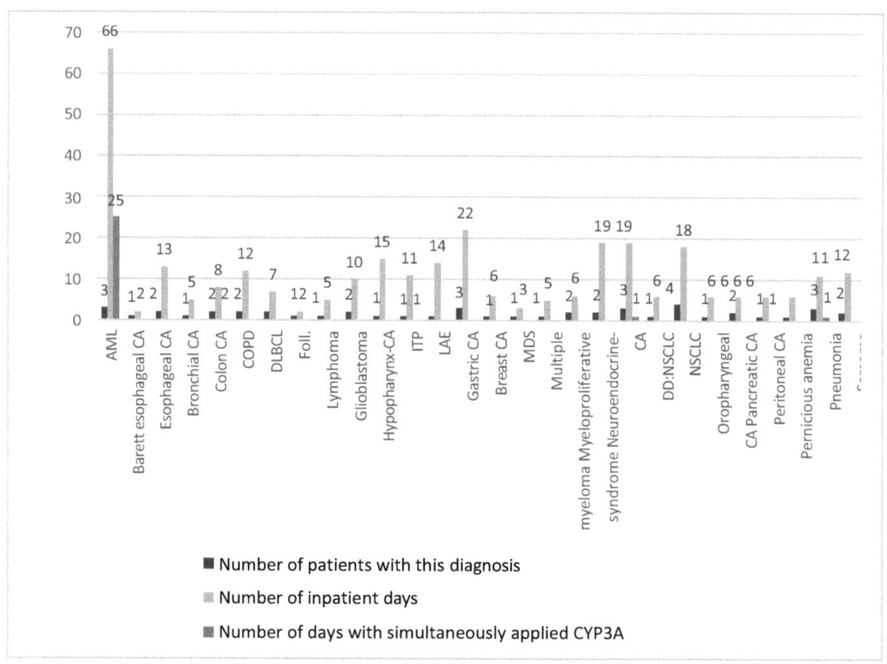

Figure 5.1: Presentation of diagnoses, their patient numbers, inpatient days and days with simultaneous CYP3A inhibitor application

It is clear that CYP3A inhibitors were applied simultaneously to AML patients on 25 days out of the total of 66 inpatient days. This results in a value of 0.379 simultaneously applied CYP3A inhibitors per day. Further diagnoses with simultaneously applied CYP3A inhibitors were SCLC (1 day with simultaneously applied CYP3A inhibitors within 11 inpatient days= 0.091 simultaneous applications of CYP3A inhibitors per day) and NSCLC (1 day with simultaneously applied CYP3A inhibitors within 19 inpatient days = 0.053 simultaneous applications of CYP3A inhibitors per day).

AML patients not only have a longer inpatient stay compared to other patients, but also have a higher number of days on which CYP3A inhibitors administered simultaneously. This puts AML patients at particular risk. In order to verify the result, the statistical significance is checked below.

5.6 Hypothesis tests

Do AML patients have a statistically significantly higher probability of simultaneous application of CYP3A inhibitors per inpatient day, in contrast to other diagnoses, or are the differences in the analyzed values due to chance? The statistical significance is analyzed using the IBM SPSS Statistics software. Since the variables are nominally scaled and the frequencies between the "AML-diagnosis patients" and the "other-diagnosis patients" are compared, the χ^2 test according to Pearson represents the best possible statistical test. The χ^2 test can make a statement as to whether the observed frequencies differ significantly from the expected frequencies, i.e. whether measures of correlation exist. As the χ^2 test can determine a significant difference between two groups of characteristics, but no effect size, further analyses such as the ϕ and the CI are carried out to quantify the effect size.

Results of the hypothesis tests

The examination was first carried out using a cross-tabulation, then as a χ^2 independence test according to Pearson and then according to the ϕ and CI in order to examine the strength of the effect of the different diagnoses. The following results were obtained:

Table 5.2: Cross-tabulation of the diagnosis AML and the other diagnoses, compared with the expected and actual number of days with simultaneous application of CYP3A inhibitors

		Days with simultaneous application:		Total
		no sim. App.	with sim. App.	
AML	Quantity	41	25	66
	Expected number	60,3	5,7	66,0
Diagnosis other	Quantity	246	2	248
	Expected number	226,7	21,3	248,0
Total	Quantity	287	27	314
	Expected number	287,0	27,0	314,0

Table 5.3: Pearson's chi-square test

	Value	df	Asymp. Sig. (2-sided)	Exact Sig. (2 pages)	Exact Sig. (1 page)
Chi-square according to Pearson	91,155[a]	1	,000		
Continuity correction [b]	86,499	1	,000		
Likelihood Quotient	73,258	1	,000		
Exact test according to Fisher				,000	,000
Number of valid cases	314				

a. 0 cells (0.0%) have an expected value less than 5. The minimum expected value is 5.68.

b. Calculated for a 2x2 table.

Since the expected number is less than 5, see Table 5.2, it can be concluded that there is an asymptotic distribution of the χ^2. (Bortz and

Lienert 2008, p. 64). The empirical, observed distribution deviates significantly from the theoretical, expected distribution, thus the null hypothesis can be rejected due to the p-value <0.05 (Bortz and Lienert 2008, p. 64). The alternative hypothesis that the data are dependent on each other and that there is therefore a correlation between the diagnosis of AML and the frequency of simultaneous application CYP3A inhibitors has therefore been confirmed. The χ^2 value according to Pearson is 91.155 and the rounded p-value is 0.000, i.e. the difference between the 2 groups is significant.

Table 5.4: Symmetrical dimensions

	Value	Approx. sig.
Phi Nominal regarding	-,539	,000
Cramer's V Nominal dimension Coefficient	,539	,000
Number of valid cases	314	

a. The null hypothesis is not accepted.

b. Assuming the null hypothesis, the asymptotic standard error is used.

The ϕ and the CI determine the correlation of the dichotomous variables and show the strength of the effect. The result is also significant here, as the expected p-values for the ϕ and CI are 0.000 and therefore the p-value of >5 is not exceeded. The days with simultaneous application of the CYP3A inhibitors of AML patients and the other diagnoses were compared. These differ significantly from each other with a strong effect, therefore a greater risk of simultaneous application of CYP3A inhibitors can be determined in the diagnosis AML. The conclusion and outlook of this scientific work are presented in the following chapter.

6. Conclusions and outlook

In this study, the questions were answered as to whether CYP3A inhibitors are applied simultaneously in routine clinical practice - namely 8.57% as measured by inpatient days (27 of 315) and 8.33% as measured by patients (4 of 48). These patients are most likely exposed to AM interactions. The frequency of simultaneously applied CYP3A inhibitors is statistically significantly higher for AML diagnoses than for other diagnoses. In AML patients, an above-average number of CYP3A inhibitors were applied simultaneously, namely 0.379 per day. The results for the two other diagnoses of NSCLC with 0.053 and SCLC with 0.091 simultaneously applied CYP3A inhibitors per inpatient day are far lower. No CYP3A inhibitors were applied simultaneously for the other diagnoses. The hypothesis tests showed that the diagnosis AML has a significantly higher probability of simultaneous application of CYP3A inhibitors within an inpatient day.

This correlation should be investigated more intensively in future studies. The analysis of further patients should focus on the diagnosis of AML and their frequency of simultaneously applied CYP3A inhibitors. For further analysis, all CYP inhibitors and also CYP inducers can be recorded, as these also interact with each other. In addition, the total adverse events of the patients should be recorded and evaluated in order to analyze whether the type of adverse events corresponds to the expected side effects caused by the AM interactions . In principle, the AM applied should help the patient and not cause unnecessary harm. Simultaneous application of CYP3A inhibitors should therefore be discouraged. A reconsideration of AM combinations in this respect is recommended in clinical routine so that sick patients are protected from interaction toxicity and do not suffer unnecessary harm. Establishing a comprehensive AM interaction warning system using software in the hospital information system would be a conceivable solution simplify the systematic checking for AM interactions. A warning message should appear in the hospital information system in the event of a potential AM interaction in order to warn hospital staff of this. At the same time, the software could offer an alternative AM that is metabolized differently. If no alternative AM is available, the doctor must decide whether the benefit outweighs the risk and the AM combination is administered anyway. In this case, delayed application may be appropriate, depending on the half-life of the active substance in the AM, or a reduction or escalation of the dose may also be considered. For the AM interaction warning system, the ethnicity and, if known, the metabolization types (poor/fast), see Chapter 2, can also be linked to the digital patient record via interfaces so that these variables also influence the dose of an AM and unnecessary side effects are reduced.

Summary

The objective of this study is the empirical investigation of the frequency of simultaneously applied CYP3A inhibitors in clinical routine. A retrospective and anonymized survey was chosen as the method. The analysis yielded the following results: 8.57% inpatient days (27 of 315) and 8.33% patients (4 of 48) were exposed to simultaneous application of CYP3A inhibitors. The frequency of simultaneously administered CYP3A inhibitors is strikingly high in patients diagnosed with AML, as an above-average number, namely 0.379 CYP3A inhibitors per day, were administered simultaneously. In comparison, NSCLC patients only 0.053 and SCLC patients only 0.091 CYP3A inhibitors simultaneously per day. The suspicion that patients with AML have a higher probability of receiving CYP3A inhibitors on inpatient days than all other patients was investigated by the hypothesis test chi-square (χ^2), the Phi coefficient (ϕ) and the Cramer's V index (CI) and to be significant. In principle, the establishment of an interaction warning system in the hospital information system would be a useful means of preventing unwanted drug interactions.

Bibliography

Bortz, Jürgen; Lienert, Gustav A. (2008): Concise statistics for clinical research. Guide for the distribution-free analysis of small samples. 3rd, updated and revised ed. Berlin, Heidelberg: Springer Medizin Verlag Heidelberg (Springer textbook).

Bühl, Achim (2008): SPSS 16. Introduction to modern data analysis. 11th, revised and expanded ed. Munich [u.a.]: Pearson Studium (Scientific tools, 7332).

Cambridgemedchemconsulting (2012): Relative Importance of CYP-450 in Drug Metabolism. Ed. by cambridgemedchemconsulting. Available online at http://www.cambridgemedchemconsulting.com/resources/ADME/cyp3a4i nhibi tion.html, last checked on 23.11.2015.

Efferth, Thomas (2007): Molekulare Pharmakologie und Toxikologie: Biologische Grundlagen von Arzneimitteln und Giften: Springer Berlin Heidelberg.

Frankfurt Hospital (2015): Preliminary analysis of the duration of inpatients.

Greiner, Christine (2009): Cytochrome P-450 isozymes. Part 1: Substrates, inducers and inhibitors. Ed. by Agate. Regensburg.

Hafner, V.; Grün, B.; Markert, C.; Czock, D.; Mikus, G.; Haefeli, W. E. (2010): Drug interactions. In: *Der Internist* 51 (3), pp. 359-69; quiz 370. DOI: 10.1007/s00108-009-2553-1.

Horton, H. Robert (2008): Biochemistry. Munich: Pearson Studium.

Ioannides, Costas; Royal Society of Chemistry (2008): Cytochromes P450: Role in the Metabolism and Toxicity of Drugs and Other Xenobiotics. Cambridge (UK): RSC Pub (p. 450).

Lücker, Peter Wolfgang; Rindt, W.; Eldon, M. (1982): Applied clinical pharmacology. Phase I trials. Berlin, Heidelberg: Springer Berlin Heidelberg (Heidelberger Taschenbücher).

Lüllmann, Heinz; Hein, Lutz; Mohr, Klaus (2010): Pharmacology and Toxicology. Understanding drug effects - targeted use of drugs; a textbook for students of medicine, pharmacy and biosciences, a source of information for doctors, pharmacists and health policy makers; 130 tables. 17th, fully revised ed. Stuttgart [et al:] Thieme.

Mutschler, Ernst (2012): Mutschler Arzneimittelwirkungen. Pharmacology - Clinical Pharmacology - Toxicology. 10th, fully revised and expanded ed. Stuttgart: Wiss. Verlagsges.

Saladax Biomedical Inc (ed.) (2014): Pharmacology. Available online at http://www.mycaretests.com/health-care-professionals/mycare-learning-center/pharmacology/, last updated on 2014, last checked on 14.01.2015.

U.S. Food and Drug Administration (2011): Drug Development and Drug Interactions: Table of Substrates, Inhibitors and Inducers. Ed. by FDA. USA. Available online at http://www.fda.gov/Drugs/DevelopmentApprovalProcess/DevelopmentResour ces/DrugInteractionsLabeling/ucm093664.htm, last checked on 23.11.2015.

Wynn, Gary H.; Oesterheld, Jessica R.; Cozza, Kelly L.; Armstrong, Scott C. (2008): Clinical Manual of Drug Interaction Principles for Medical Practice. The P450 System. Arlington: American Psychiatric Pub.

List of abbreviations

AM Pharmaceuticals

AML Acute myeloid leukemia AUC Area under the curve

CA Carcinoma

CI Cramer's V-index

CL Clearance

C_{max} Maximum concentration C_{min} Minimum concentration

CRF Case Report Form CYP3A Cytochrome P-3A CYP-450 Cytochrome P-450 H0 Null hypothesis

H1 Alternative hypothesis

NSCLC Non-Small-Cell-Lung-Cancer SCLC Small-Cell-Lung-Cancer

$t½$ Terminal elimination half-life χ^2-test Chi-square test

ϕ Phi-coefficient

Appendix

The CRF (Excel) and the database (SPSS) have been uploaded separately or burned to CD due to their size.

CYP3A- Inhibitoren

Strong Inhibitors(2) ≥ 5-fold increase in AUC or > 80% decrease in CL (Clearance)

- Boceprevir: Victrelis
- Clarithromycin: Clarilind, Clarithrobeta, Klacid, Helicomp
- Conivaptan: Vaprisol (nur USA)
- Grapefruit Juice
- Indinavir: Crixivan
- Itraconazole: Itracol, Itraconazol, Itraconbeta, Itraderm, Sempera, Siros, Sporanox,
- Ketoconazole: Fungoral, Ket Med, Ketozolin, Nizoral, Terzolin
- Lopinavir/Ritonavir: Kaletra/Norvir
- Mibefradil: Posicor (USA)
- Nefazodone: Dutonin, Nefadar, Serzone
- Nelfinavir: Viracept
- Posaconazole: Noxafil
- Saquinavir: Invirase
- Telaprevir: Incivo
- Telithromycin: Ketek
- Voriconazole: Vfend

Moderate inhibitors(3) ≥ 2 but < 5-fold increase in AUC or 50-80% decrease in CL

- Amprenavir: Telzir
- Aprepitant: Emend
- Atazanavir: Reyataz
- Ciprofloxacin: Cipro, Ciloxan, Ciprobay, Cilodex, Ciprobeta, Cirpodoc, Ciprodura, Ciprofat, Ciproflox, Gyracip, Infectocipro, Keciflox, Panotile, Cipro-Q, Ciprovert
- Darunavir/Ritonavir: Prezista/Norvir
- Diltiazem: Dilzem, DiltaHexal, Dilti, Diltiagamma, Diltiazem,
- Erythromycin: Infectomycin, Aknefug El, Eryaknen, Erycinum, Eryhexal, Erythro, Erythrocin, Inderm, Isotrexin, Paediathrocin, Stiemycine, Zineryt, Aknederm, Erydermec, Sanasepton
- Fluconazole: Diflucan, Flucobeta, Flucoderm, Flucolich, Fluconazol, Flunazul
- Fosamprenavir: Telzir

Erstellt von Diana Dmytrow am 20.01.15

- grapefruit juice
- Imatinib: Glivec
- Verapamil: Cordichin (Kombipräparat), Isoptin, Tarka (Kombipräparat), Vera, Veragamma, Verahexal, Vera Lich, Veramex, Verapamil, Veratide (Kombipräparat), VeroptinStada, Falicard, Veroptin

Weak inhibitors(4) $\geq$ 1.25 but < 2-fold increase in AUC or 20-50% decrease in CL

- Alprazolam: Tafil, Cassadan
- Amiodarone: Amiodaron, Cordarex, Amiodura, Amiogamma, Amiohexal, Cordarone,
- Amlodipine: Exforge, Amlo-Q-Besilat, Amlobesilat, Amlobeta, Amliclair, Amlodigamma, Amlodoc, Amlolich, Amlo Tad, Amparo, Dafiro (Kombipräparat), Exforge (Kombipräparat), Norvasc, Ramipril (Kombipräparat), Sevikar (Kombipräparat), Tonotec (Kombipräparat), Twynsta (Kombipräparat), Vocado (Kombipräparat)
- Atorvastatin: Atorgamma, Atoris, Lipitor, Sortis, Atorva-Q, Atorvastatin
- Bicalutamide: Bicalutamid, Androcal, Bica-Q, Bicadex, Bicalut, Bicalutin, Bicamed, Casodex, Eurobicalutamid
- Cilostazol: Pletal
- Cimetidine: Cim Lich, Cimetidin, H2-Blocker, Tagamet
- Cyclosporine: Cicloral, Ciclosporin, Ciqorin, Deximune, Sandimmun
- Fluoxetine: Fluoxgamma, Fluoxelich, Fluox Puren, Fluoxet
- Fluvoxamine: Fevarin, Fluvoxamin, Fluvoxamin Neurax
- Ginkgo: Bioxera (Kombipräparat), Btf Geria (Kombipräparat), Cereginkgo H, Ceres Ginkgo Dryopt, DS Concept Angio Cardial, Evisko Ginkgo, Ginkgo Biloba, Ginkgo Bioxera, Ginkgo Com Pflueger, Ginkgo Immergrün, Ginkgorell, Ginkgo Schuck, Homeda Ginkgo, Lm Ginkgo, Metaginkgo (Kombipräparat), RT Arterio 3 (Kombipräparat), Retroplex (Kombipräparat), Rosskastanie Komplex (Kombipräparat), Similex Ginkgo, Spiraphan (Kombipräparat), Stella Komplex (Kombipräparat), Weissdorn Ginkgo (Kombipräparat), Wuweizi und Ginkgo
- Goldenseal (Hydrastis Canadensis): -
- Isoniazid: Isozid, Tebesium-S, Tebesium, Iso Eremfat
- Nilotinib: Tasigna
- Oral contraceptives: (Levonorgestrel Kombipräparate) 28 Mini, Asumate, Cleogyn, Cyclo Progynova, Erlibelle, Erlidona, Estelle,

Ethinylestr, Evaluna, Fem 7, Femigoa, Femigyne, Femikadin, Femranette, Glorianna, Gravistat, Illina, Jaydess, Junonia beta, Kleodina, Klimonorm, Leanova, Leios, Leona Hexal, Levina Stada, Levomin, Liana, Logynon, Luisa, Maexeni, Microgynon, Microginon, Microlut, Minisiston, Miranova, Mirena, Monostep, Novastep, Oestronara, Ovoplex, Pidana, Postinor, Stediril, Swingo, Trigoa, Trigynon, Trinordiol, Triquilar, Trisiston, Unofem, Wellnara, Brintesia beta, Cyclo Oestrogenal, Femranette, Lalydia, Microlut, Minisiston, Triette, (Ethinylestradiol Kombipräparate) Aida, Aidulan, Alessia, Amelie, Amicette, Angiletta, Aristelle, Attempta, Beatrice, Belara, Belinda, Bella, Bellissima, Bilmon, Biviol, Bonadea, Bonita, Cedia, Chariva, Chloee, Cilest, Circlet, Cleogyn, Conceplan, Cyproderm, Daylette, Desmin, Desofemine, Diane 35, Dienogenance, Dienovel, Drosfemine, Drospifem, Eliza, Enriqa, Ergalea, Eve, Evra, Famina, Femodene, Femovan, Finic, Gabrielle, Gracial, Helen, Illina, Jennifer, Juliane, Juliette, Kosima, Ladonna, Lamiva, Lamuna, Laviola, Layaisa, Layanina, Leanova, Leona, Lilia, Lisette, Lovelle, Luvyna, Lysandra, Madinance, Madinette, Maexeni, Maitalon, Marvelon, Maxim, Mayra, Mercilon, Minette, Minulet, Mona, Morea, Munalea, Mywy, Neo Eunomin, Novial, Nuvaring, Ovoplex, Petibelle, Pink Luna, Previva, Sibilla, Sidretella, Solera, Starletta, Stediril, Stella, Susette, Swingo, Synphase, Trigoa, Trinordiol, Trinovum, Valette, Velafee, Velvet, Verana, Veyanne, Veya, Violette, Yara, Yasmin, Yasminelle, Yaz, Yiznell, Aricia beta, Belanca, Brintesia, Eufem, Issoria, Lalydia, Laynes, Lonicera, Pramino, Synphase, Synphasec, Triette, Vatrice

- Ranitidine: Ranitic, Junizac, Ranibeta, Ranidura, Raniberl, Ranicux, Raniprotect
- Ranolazine: Ranexa
- Tipranavir/Ritonavir: Aptivus/Norvir
- Zileuton: Zileuton

Quellen: FDA, Ifap-Liste und Internet Google-Suche – deutsche Handelsnamen - Stand 13.01.2015

Erstellt von Diana Dmytrow am 20.01.15

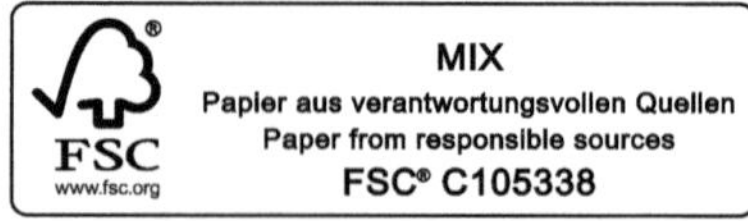

Printed by Books on Demand GmbH, Norderstedt / Germany